The Slow Cooker Cookbook

The Ultimate Healthy Slow Cooker Cookbook Including Deliciously Satisfying Meals that are Prepared Quickly and Cooked Slowly. Bonus Includes Low-Carb, Keto, Vegan, Vegetarian, and Mediterranean Crockpot Recipes!

The Vibrant Chef

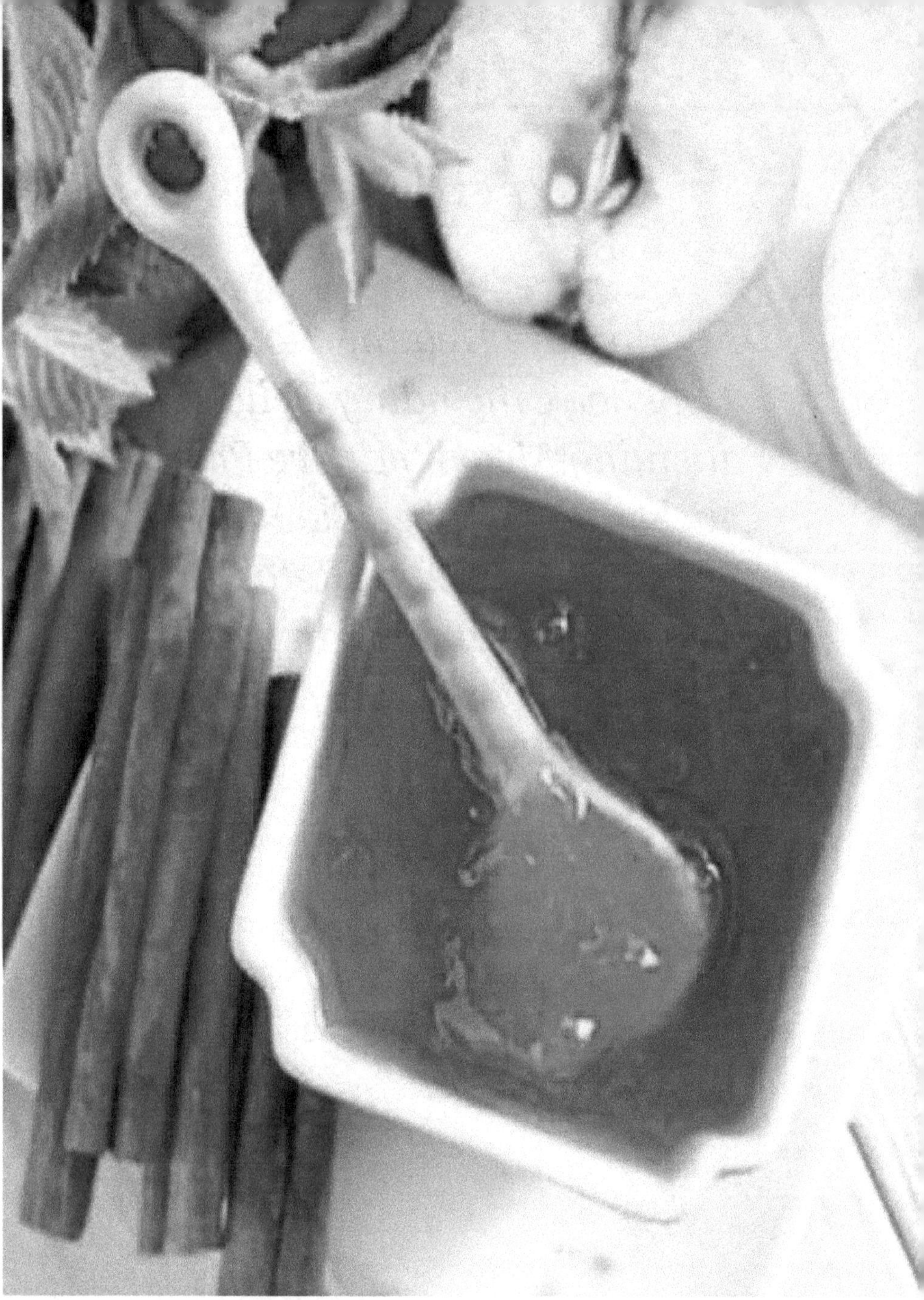

Table of Contents

Introduction

book, we will show you the importance of having a slow cooker in your life. It is a complete guide for you.

A slow cooker, or crock-pot, is an electronic appliance used to simmer the food at a lower temperature than other cooking methods. Why you should choose the slow cooker cooking method? Nowadays our life is so busy that we don't have enough time to spend in the kitchen and make delicious dishes. The slow cooker has made our lives easier. It produces tasty recipes and also saves money and time.

The slow cooker process has to be started long before eating time because it takes a long time to produce healthy and tasty food.

Foods you can cook in a slow cooker include:

- Meat and poultry
- Beans
- Fish

- Corn
- Stuffing
- Porridge
- Jams
- Broths
- Desserts

Foods you should never put in a slow cooker include:

- Milk
- Cream
- Cheese
- Yogurt
- Pasta
- Rice
- Boneless chicken
- Couscous

Using a slow cooker does not require expert cooking skills. Every slow cooker has its own manual which you should read before trying a recipe. It is very simple to use a slow cooker.

Step 1:

First of all, the slow cooker requires a little preparation. You simply need to chop the vegetables and meat into small chunks and pre-heat the cooker.

Step 2:

If you are cooking root vegetables, place them at the bottom of the cooker because they take a long time to cook. If you are preparing meat or poultry, place your food on the top and then add liquid so the food doesn't dry out.

Step 3:

One you have added all the ingredients, simply set the temperature and timer of the cooker. The temperature is kept low for a longer cooking period and high for a shorter cooking period.

After you have served your food, remove the pot from the slow cooker and fill it with hot soapy water. Then leave to soak and dry the pot completely before setting back in the cooker.

Healthy

Slow cookers are great for creating healthier meals. This is because they rarely require oils or fats in the cooking process. Standard cooking methods eliminate the vitamins and minerals from the food. But a slow cooker keeps the food juicy and preserves a lot of vitamins and minerals.

Flavor

Slow cookers produce delicious food full of flavor. When the food is left to stew for hours the meat becomes more tender and the sauces richer as their full flavor is released.

Quick and Easy

Cooking a healthy meal is simplified by using a slow cooker. You simply put the ingredients into the cooker and set it to cook. You can cook your meal throughout the day without henever you wish.

Poultry

Servings: 8

Preparation Time: 5 hours 10 minutes

Per Serving: Calories 565 Fat 21.8 g Carbohydrates 1.7 g Sugar 0.6 g Protein 84.8 g Cholesterol 260 mg

Ingredients:

- 1/2 cup green onion, sliced
- 2 packets taco seasoning
- 2 cups chicken stock
- 16 chicken thighs, bone- in and skin-on
- 1/2 tsp red pepper flakes

Procedure:

1. First, add stock and half the taco seasoning to a crock pot. Stir well to blend.
2. Then place chicken thighs in the crock pot and sprinkle remaining seasoning on top of chicken.
3. Now cover and cook on low for 5 hours.
4. Garnish with red pepper flakes and green onions.

Servings: 8

Preparation Time: 1 hour

Per Serving: Calories: 387 Fat: 12g Carbs: 7g

Ingredients:

- 2 Onions, thinly sliced
- 4 garlic cloves, minced
- 12 Boneless Skinless Chicken Thighs
- 2 Cups Salsa Verde (use Trader Joe's)

Procedure:

1. Heat oven to 350F.
2. In a dutch oven or glass baking dish arrange chicken thighs in a single layer. Top with salsa, onions, and garlic.
3. Cover and bake for 60-90 minutes or until chicken is fully cooked and onions are translucent.
4. Shred chicken (you can use 2 forks).
5. Once chicken has been shredded, use a wooden spoon to combine shredded chicken and juices.

Servings: 6

Preparation Time: 6 hours

Per Serving: Calories: 326 Fat: 30g Carbs: 60g

Ingredients:

- 1 tablespoon red wine vinegar
- Juice of ½ medium lemon
- ⅓ cup water
- 1 teaspoon dried oregano leaves
- ½ teaspoon salt
- ½ teaspoon pepper
- 3 tablespoons olive oil
- 2 lb boneless skinless chicken breast
- 1 onion, chopped
- 2 cloves garlic, minced

Tzatziki Sauce:

- Salt and pepper, to taste
- Juice of ½ medium lemon
- 1 tablespoon extra-virgin olive oil

- 2 to 3 cloves garlic, minced
- 2 cups plain greek yogurt
- 1 tablespoon white wine vinegar
- 1 teaspoon dried dill weed
- 1 teaspoon dried oregano leaves

Procedure:

1. Spay a slow cooker with cooking spray. Add the chicken to the slow cooker. In a small bowl combine onion, garlic, oregano, salt, pepper, olive oil, red wine vinegar, lemon juice, and water. Pour over chicken.
2. Cook on low for 6-8 hours or high for 4-6.
3. To make the sauce: In a medium bowl combine greek yogurt, cucumber, garlic, white wine vinegar, dried dill week, dried oregano.
4. Salt and pepper to taste and add lemon juice and drizzle olive oil on top.
5. Refrigerate for 30 minutes to let the flavors blend.
6. Prepare chicken on warm greek pita bread with desired vegetables and sauce on top.

Servings: 4

Preparation Time: 4 hours

Per Serving: Calories: 237 Fat: 2g Carbs: 40g

Ingredients:

- 2 tablespoons corn starch
- 2 boneless, skinless chicken breasts
- 1-2 teaspoons lemon zest optional
- 1/2 cup liquid honey
- 1/2 cup fresh squeezed lemon juice
- 2 tablespoons low sodium soy sauce
- 1/2 teaspoon salt
- 1 pinch of pepper
- 1/4 cup low sodium chicken broth

Procedure:

1. In a 2.5-4 quart slow cooker, combine broth, honey, juice, soy sauce, salt, pepper and corn starch with a whisk until combined.

4. If sauce is thin, mix another 1 tablespoon water and 1 tablespoon corn starch and stir into the sauce to thicken further. If desired, adjust seasonings and add lemon zest if desired (it will make it very lemony!).

5. Serve over hot cooked rice.

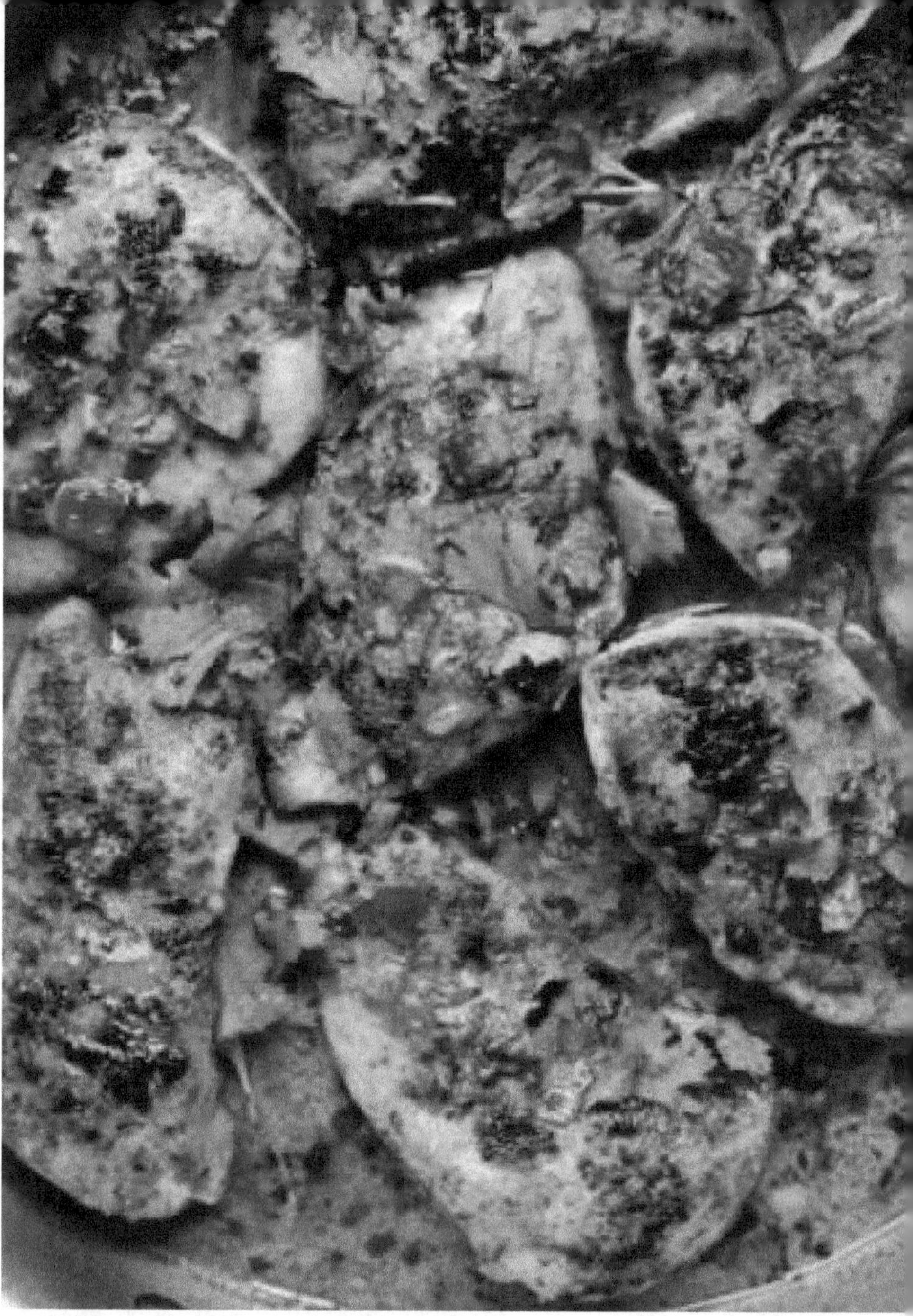

Servings: 4

Preparation Time: 6 hours

Per Serving: Calories: 237 Fat: 2g Carbs: 40g

Ingredients:

- 2 serrano (or jalapeno) peppers, minced (optional)
- 1/2 cup low-sodium chicken broth
- 1 pound chicken breasts
- 1 (15 oz) can no salt added black beans, drained and rinsed
- 1 cup corn kernals (fresh, frozen or canned)
- 2 Tbsp fresh lime juice
- 1 Tbsp cumin
- Optional toppings for serving: salsa, cheese, avocado
- 1 medium red bell pepper, diced
- 1/2 cup onion, diced
- 1/4 cup cilantro, finely chopped

1. Add all ingredients to slow cooker.
2. Stir to combine and cook on low for 4-6 hours.
3. Remove chicken, shred, return to pot, stir and serve.
4. Place all ingredients in a large ziploc bag and freeze fla
5. Prior to cooking, defrost over night in the refrigerator or under cold running water.
6. Dump contents into the crockpot. Add a little bit of water to the bag, shake it around and add to crockpot t help get some of the cilantro out if it sticks to the bag.
7. Cook on low 4-6 hours.
8. Shred chicken breasts and serve over rice, as is or in tortillas.

Servings: 6

Preparation Time: 8 hours

Per Serving: Calories: 338; Total Fat: 15g; Saturated Fat: 3g; Cholesterol: 127mg; Sodium: 480mg; Total Carbohydrates: 19g; Fiber: 1g; Protein: 32g

Ingredients:

- 1 teaspoon dried oregano
- ½ teaspoon salt, plus more for seasoning
- ¼ teaspoon freshly ground black pepper, plus more for
- 1 large onion, halved and thinly sliced
- ¼ cup olive oil
- 2 tablespoons fresh lemon juice
- 2 pounds boneless, skinless chicken thighs, trimmed of excess fat
- 2 teaspoons garlic powder
- seasoning
- 6 pita breads, warmed
- Tzatziki sauce, for serving

- chopped lettuce, tomatoes, red bell peppers, and cucumbers

Procedure:

1. Put the chicken and onion in the slow cooker.
2. In a small bowl, whisk together the olive oil, lemon juice, garlic powder, oregano, salt, and pepper.
3. Pour the mixture over the chicken and onion and toss to coat.
4. Cover and cook on low for 8 hours, or until the chicken is tender.
5. Transfer the chicken to a cutting board. Shred the chicken with two forks, then return it to the slow cooker. Stir.
6. Season with additional salt and pepper, if needed. Serv the chicken and onions with pita breads, and pass the tzatziki sauce and chopped vegetables, if desired.

Servings: 5

Preparation Time: 6 hours 15 minutes

Per Serving: Calories: 638; Total Fat: 38g; Saturated Fat: 21g; Cholesterol: 257mg; Sodium: 593mg; Total Carbohydrates: 6g; Fiber: 2g; Protein: 72g

Ingredients:

- 1 (13.5-ounce) can coconut milk, stirred
- 2 tablespoons Sriracha sauce
- 1 tablespoon Thai garlic chili paste
- 1 tablespoon tamari or low-sodium soy sauce
- 1 teaspoon dried basil 3 to 4 pounds chicken drumsticks
- Steamed rice, for serving (optional)
- Chopped fresh cilantro, for garnish (optional)

Procedure:

1. Combine the coconut milk, Sriracha sauce, Thai garlic chili paste, and tamari in the slow cooker.
2. Stir to combine.

the chicken drumsticks.

4. Add the now skinless chicken drumsticks to the slow cooker, nestling them into the sauce.
5. Cover and cook on low for 6 hours.
6. If desired, serve the chicken and sauce over rice and garnish with cilantro.

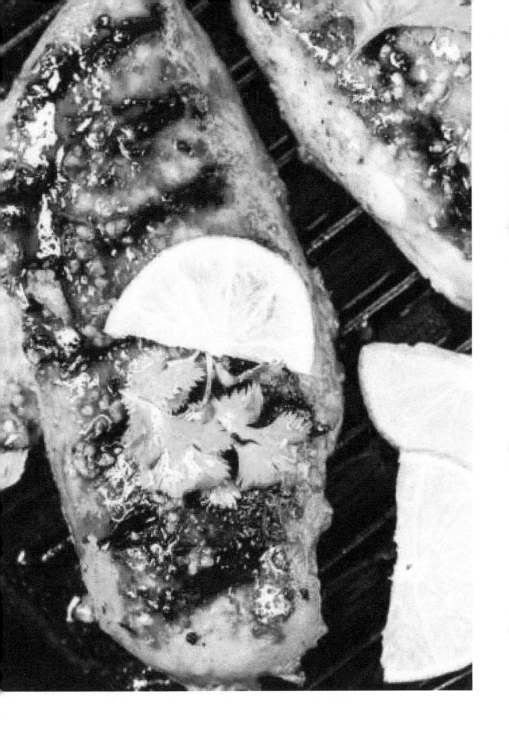

Servings: 4

Preparation Time: 6 hours

Per Serving: Calories: 315; Total Fat: 9g; Saturated Fat: 2g; Cholesterol: 190mg; Sodium: 2,254mg; Total Carbohydrates 10g; Fiber: 1g; Protein: 48g

Ingredients:

- 2 pounds boneless, skinless chicken thighs, trimmed of excess fat
- ½ cup tamari or low-sodium soy sauce
- ¼ cup fresh lime juice
- 1 tablespoon Worcestershire sauce
- 2 garlic cloves, minced
- 1 tablespoon brown sugar
- ½ teaspoon freshly ground black pepper
- 2 tablespoons cornstarch
- 2 tablespoons water

1. Put the chicken thighs in the slow cooker.
2. In a medium bowl, whisk together the tamari, lime juice, Worcestershire sauce, garlic, brown sugar, and pepper. Pour the mixture over the chicken.
3. Cover and cook on low for 6 hours, or until the chicken is tender.
4. Turn the slow cooker to high.
5. In a small bowl, whisk together the cornstarch and water.
6. Stir the cornstarch slurry into the liquid in the slow cooker.
7. Let the sauce thicken for 10 minutes.
8. Serve the chicken with the sauce.

Servings: 6

Preparation Time: 6 hours 15 minutes

Per Serving: Calories: 251; Total Fat: 7g; Saturated Fat: 2g
Cholesterol: 127mg;Sodium: 1,199mg; Total Carbohydrates:
13g; Fiber: 2g; Protein: 33g

Ingredients:

- ½ cup oyster sauce
- ¼ cup tamari or low-sodium soy sauce
- ¼ cup (packed) brown sugar
- 2 tablespoons cornstarch
- 2 tablespoons water
- 1 (16-ounce) package frozen broccoli florets
- 1 teaspoon toasted sesame oil
- 1 cup chicken broth
- 1 teaspoon garlic powder
- 2 pounds boneless, skinless chicken thighs, trimmed of excess fat and cut into bite-size pieces

Procedure:

1. Combine the chicken broth, oyster sauce, tamari, brown sugar, sesame oil, and garlic powder in the slow cooker.

2. Whisk until smooth.

3. Add the chicken pieces and stir to coat with the sauce.

4. Cover and cook on low for 6 hours, or until the chicken is tender.

5. Remove the lid and turn the cooker to high.

6. Make a cornstarch slurry by whisking the cornstarch and water together in a small bowl.

7. Add the slurry to the liquid in the slow cooker and whisk until dissolved.

8. Pour the broccoli into a colander.

9. Run hot water over the broccoli until it's warmed through.

10. Shake off the excess water and then stir the broccoli into the slow cooker.

11. Cover and cook on high for 10 minutes, or until the broccoli is cooked through and the sauce is thickened by the cornstarch.

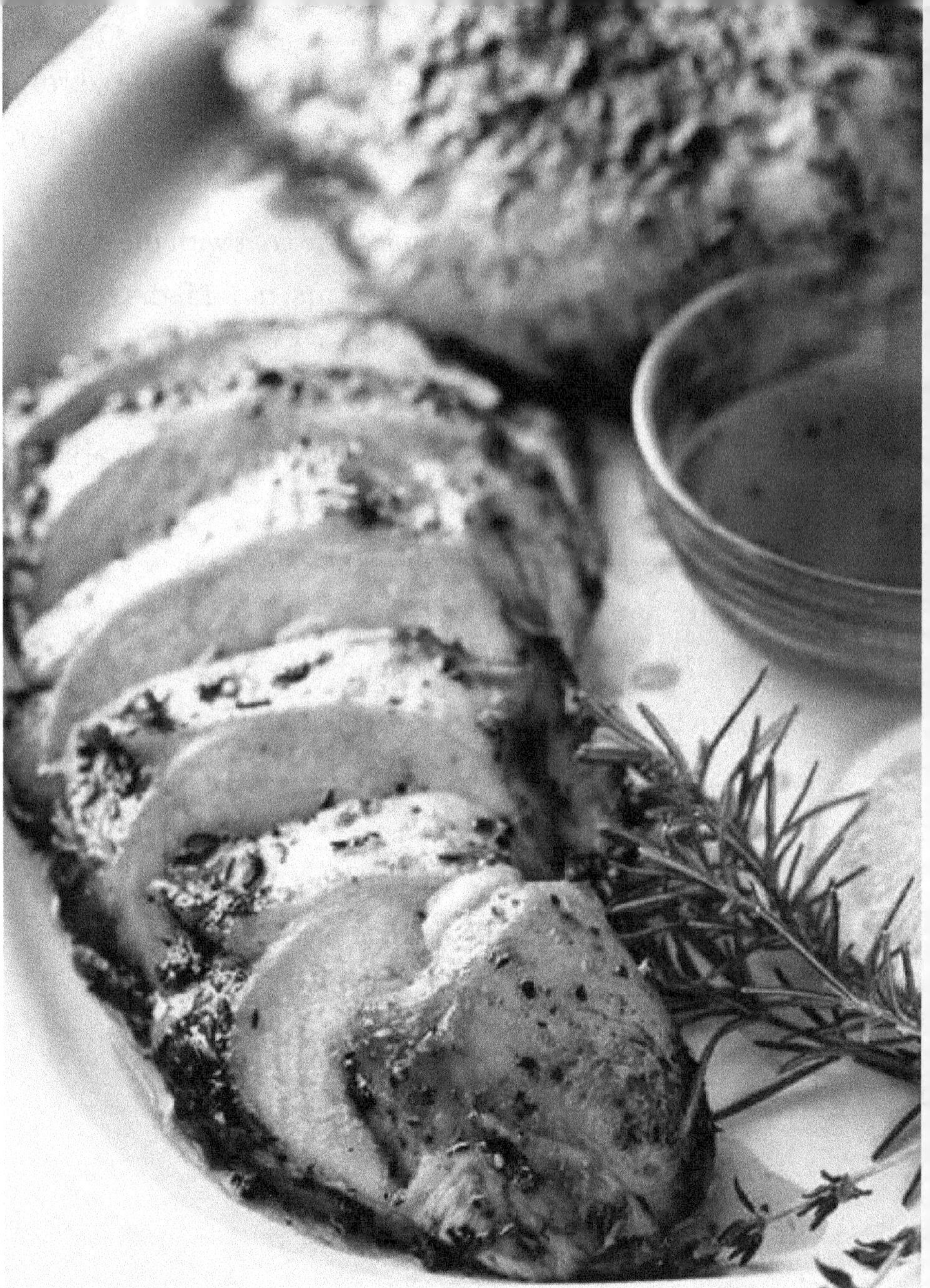

Servings: 8

Preparation Time: 3 hours 40 minutes

Per Serving: 246 calories, 19.7g protein, 18.4g carbohydrates, 10.7g fat, 1g fiber, 72mg cholesterol, 1512mg sodium, 379mg potassium.

Ingredients:

- 2 teaspoons smoked paprika
- 1 teaspoon salt
- 2 cups of water
- 2-pounds turkey breast, skinless, boneless
- 6 tablespoons of liquid honey
- 2 teaspoons chili powder
- 6 tablespoons butter

Procedure:

1. Sprinkle the turkey breast with salt, smoked paprika, and chili powder.
2. Put the turkey in the slow cooker, add water, and close the lid.

3. Cook the meal on High for 3 hours.
4. Then drain water and sprinkle the turkey breast with butter and liquid honey.
5. Carefully mix the turkey breast and cook it on High for 30 minutes.

Servings: 8

Preparation Time: 7 hours 10 minutes

Per Serving: 280 calories, 30.1g protein, 23.4g carbohydrates, 7.7g fat, 3.7g fiber, 88mg cholesterol, 93mg sodium, 515mg potassium.

Ingredients:

- 2 teaspoons peppercorns
- 2 tablespoons dried dill
- 10 oz fresh figs, chopped
- 28 oz chicken fillet, chopped
- 2 cups of water

Procedure:

1. First, put all ingredients in the slow cooker.
2. Close the lid and cook the meal on Low for 7 hours.

Servings: 8

Preparation Time: 2 hours 40 minutes

Per Serving: 275 calories, 27.2g protein, 3.9g carbohydrates 18.1g fat, 0.9g fiber, 103mg cholesterol, 240mg sodium, 378mg potassium.

Ingredients:

- 1 cup cream
- 2 teaspoons ground black pepper
- 4 tomatoes, chopped
- 20 oz ground turkey
- 2 cups Monterey Jack cheese, shredded

Procedure:

1. First, put ground turkey in the slow cooker.
2. Then add cheese, cream, and ground black pepper.

4. Then carefully mix the mixture and transfer in the serving bowls.
5. Top the ground turkey with chopped tomatoes.

Servings: 8

Preparation Time: 2 hours 15 minutes

Per Serving: 236 calories, 15.3g protein, 10.5g carbohydrates, 13.7g fat, 1.1g fiber, 0mg cholesterol, 1198mg sodium, 145mg potassium.

Ingredients:

- 2 tablespoons dried sage
- 2 teaspoons salt
- 2 teaspoons olive oil
- 2-pounds chicken sausages
- 2 cups tomato juice

Procedure:

1. First, heat the olive oil in the skillet well.
2. Then add chicken sausages and roast them for 1 minut per side on high heat.
3. Then transfer the chicken sausages in the slow cooker.
4. Now add all remaining ingredients and close the lid.
5. Cook the chicken sausages on High for 2 hours.

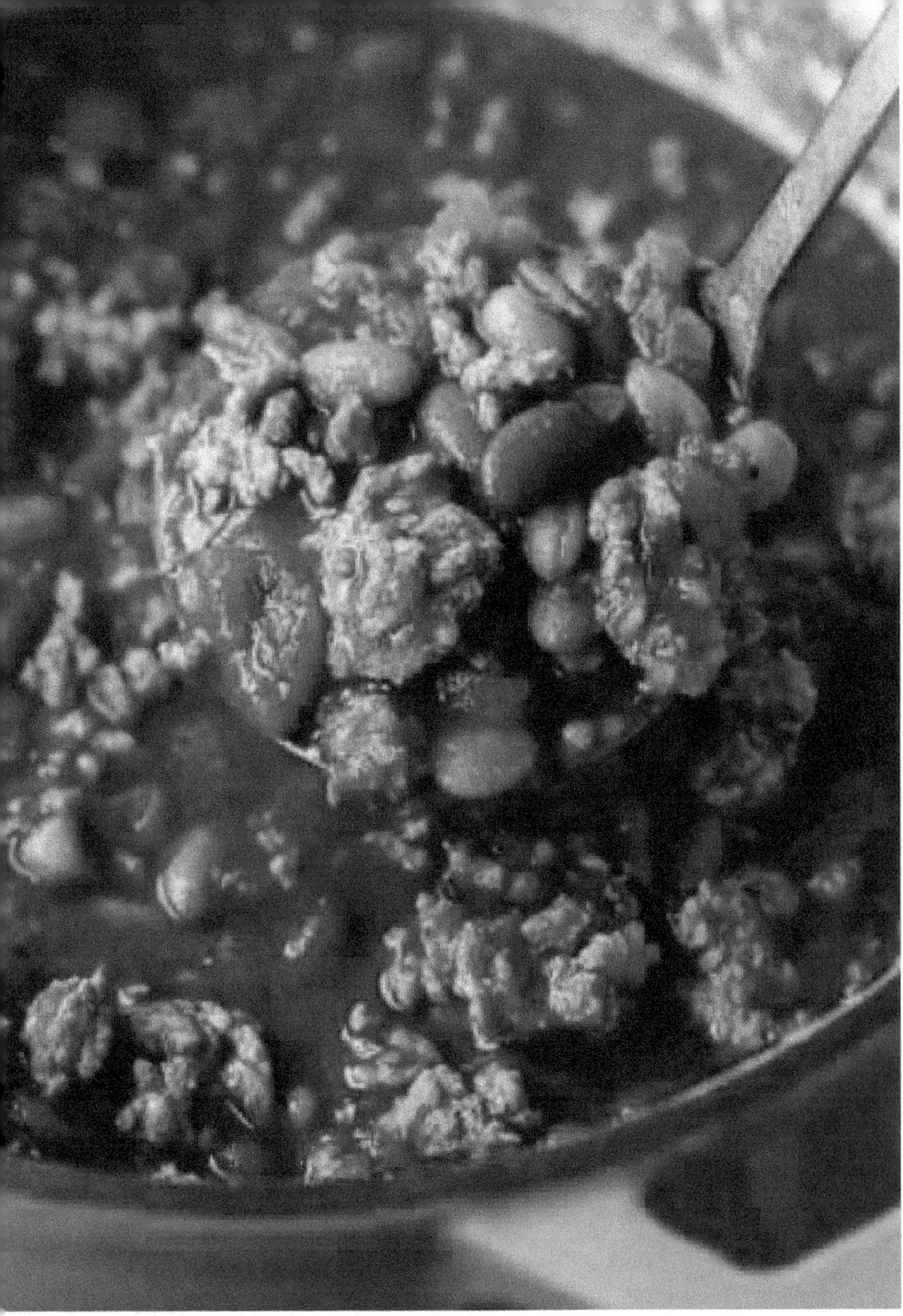

Seafood

Servings: 8

Preparation Time: 2 hours 40 minutes

Per Serving: Calories 200 Fat 7.7 g Carbohydrates 4.6 g Sugar 0 g Protein 26 g Cholesterol 239 mg

Ingredients:

- 2 Tbsp curry paste
- 30 oz water
- 60 oz coconut milk
- 2 lb shrimp
- 1/2 cup fresh cilantro, chopped
- 4 tsp lemon garlic seasoning

Procedure:

1. First add coconut milk, cilantro, lemon garlic seasoning, curry paste, and water to a crock pot and stir well.
2. Then cover and cook on high for 2 hours.
3. Now add shrimp, cover and cook for 30 minutes longer.

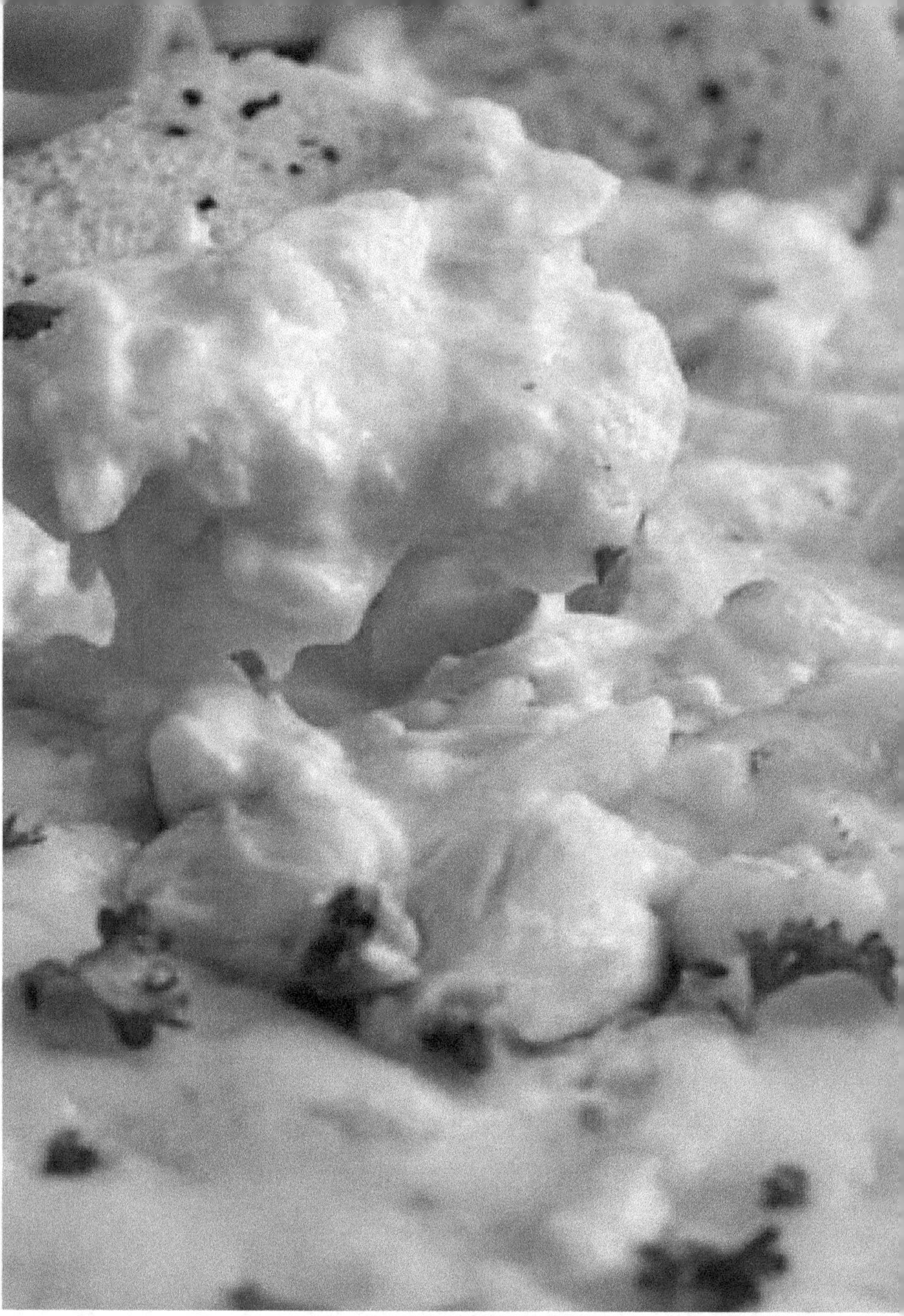

Servings: 24

Preparation Time: 3 hours 10 minutes

Per Serving: Calories 53 Fat 4.2 g Carbohydrates 2.4 g Sugar 0.6 g Protein 1.8 g Cholesterol 12 mg

Ingredients:

- 2 Tbsp onion, chopped
- 8 oz cream cheese
- 1 tsp hot sauce
- 8 oz imitation crab meat
- 1 tsp paprika
- 1/4 cup walnuts, chopped

Procedure:

1. First, place all ingredients, except paprika and walnuts, in a crock pot and stir well.
2. Then sprinkle over the paprika and walnuts.
3. Cover and cook on low for 3 hours.
4. Stir well and serve.

Tempting Lemon Butter Tilapia

Servings: 8

Preparation Time: 2 hours 10 minutes

Per Serving: Calories 112 Fat 6.7 g Carbohydrates 3.8 g Sugar 2.3 g Protein 10 g Cholesterol 37 mg

Ingredients:

- 1 1/2 cup fresh lemon juice
- 24 asparagus spear
- 8 tilapia fillets
- 1/2 tsp lemon pepper seasoning
- 4 Tbsp butter, divided

Procedure:

1. First, prepare four large sheets of aluminum foil.
2. Then place a fish fillet on each sheet.
3. Sprinkle lemon pepper seasoning and lemon juice on top of fish fillets.
4. Then add 1/2 tablespoon of butter on top of each fillet.

7. Repeat with the remaining fish fillets.
8. Place fish fillet packets in a crock pot.
9. Cover and cook on high for 2 hours.

Servings: 12

Preparation Time: 4 hours 15 minutes

Per Serving: Calories: 102 Fat: 1g Carbohydrates: 4.6g

Ingredients:

- 1 cup feta cheese
- 2 pounds shell clams
- 1 cup white wine
- 1 1/3 cup fresh lemon juice
- 4 teaspoons garlic powder
- 1/4 cup tea seed oil

Procedure:

1. First, mix together white wine, tea seed oil and lemon juice in a bowl.
2. Then microwave for 1 minute and stir well to refrigerat for 1 day.

4. Cover and cook on LOW for about 4 hours.

5. Stir in the feta cheese well and dish out to serve hot.

Servings: 8

Preparation Time:5 hours 20 minutes

Per Serving: Calories: 163 Fat: 7.1g Protein 24 g

Ingredients:

- 2 tablespoons fresh lemon juice
- 2 tablespoons tea seed oil
- 2 pounds tilapia fillets
- 2 tablespoons avocado mayonnaise
- ¼ teaspoon dried thyme
- Salt and black pepper, to taste
- ½ cup Pecorino Romano cheese, grated

Procedure:

1. First, mix together all the ingredients except tilapia fillets in a bowl.
2. Then arrange the tilapia fillets in the crock pot and pour in the mixture.
3. Now cover and cook on LOW for about 5 hours.
4. Dish out in a serving platter and immediately serve.

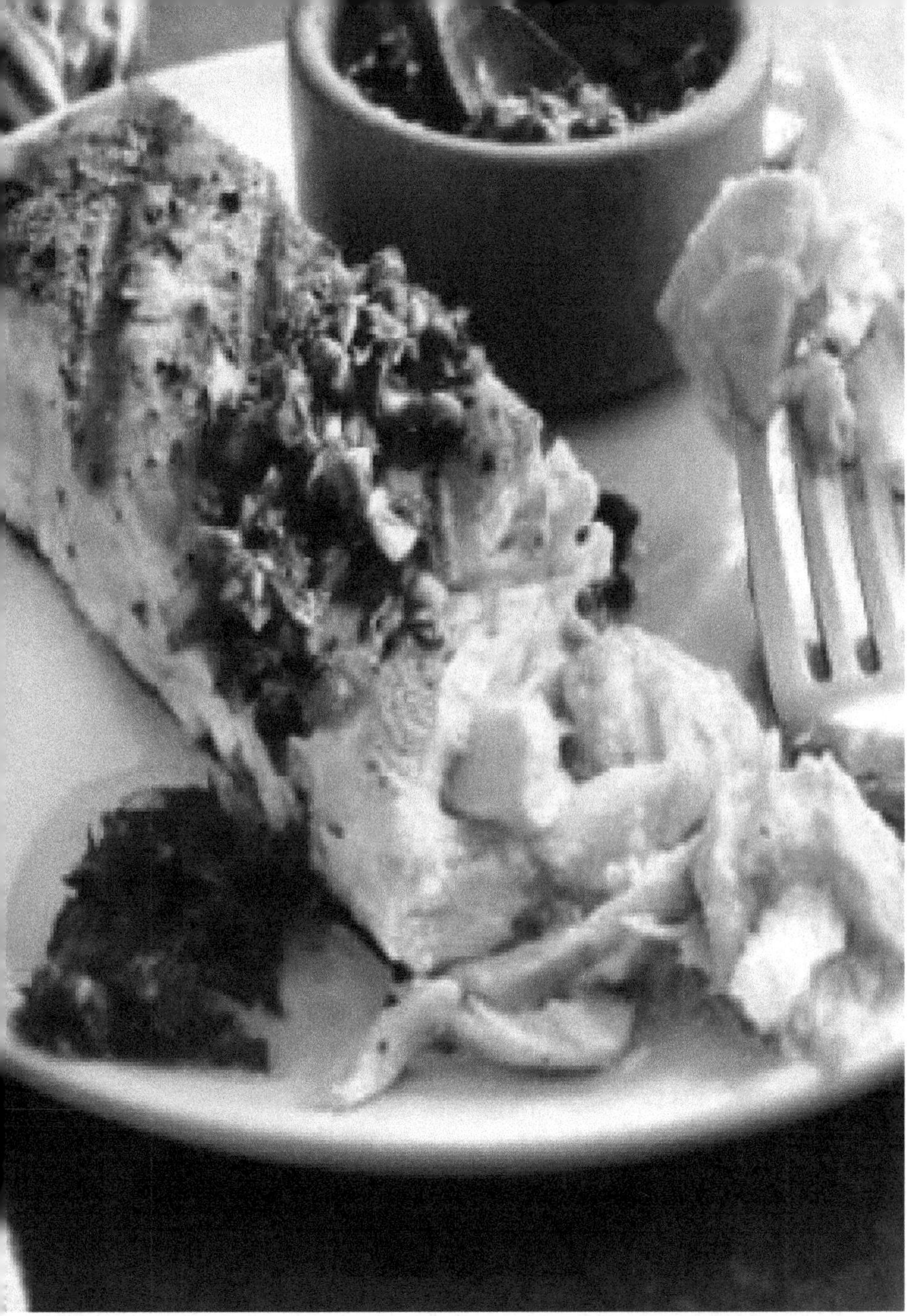

Servings: 12

Preparation Time: 5 hours 30 minutes

Per Serving: Calories: 191 Fat: 11.7 g Carbohydrates: 0.2 g

Ingredients:

- 48-ounce salmon fillets
- Salt and black pepper, to taste
- 6 tablespoons fresh parsley, minced
- 1/2 teaspoon ginger powder
- 4 tablespoons olive oil

Procedure:

1. First, mix together all the ingredients except salmon fillets in a bowl.
2. Then marinate salmon fillets in this mixture for about hour.
3. Transfer the marinated salmon fillets into the crock pc and cover the lid.
4. Cook on LOW for about 5 hours and dish out to serve hot.

Servings: 4

Preparation Time: 1 hour 45 minutes

Per Serving: 254 calories, 25.3g protein, 13.8g carbohydrates, 11g fat, 1.1g fiber, 137mg cholesterol, 234mg sodium, 78mg potassium.

Ingredients:

- 2 tablespoons coconut oil
- 1/2 cup of water
- 4 cod fillets
- 2 eggs, beaten
- 2/3 cup breadcrumbs
- 2 teaspoons ground black pepper

Procedure:

1. First, cut the cod fillets into medium sticks and sprinkle with ground black pepper.
2. Then dip the fish in the beaten egg and coat in the breadcrumbs.

4. Add coconut oil and fish sticks.

5. Cook the meal on High for 1.5 hours.

Servings: 12

Preparation Time: 7 hours 15 minutes

Per Serving: 158 calories, 9.5g protein, 18.6g carbohydrates, 5g fat, 1.3g fiber, 19mg cholesterol, 524mg sodium, 191mg potassium.

Ingredients:

- 2 teaspoons salt
- 2 tablespoons fresh dill
- 2 teaspoons olive oil
- 14 oz. yeast dough
- 2 tablespoons cream cheese
- 16 oz. salmon fillet, chopped
- 2 onions, diced

Procedure:

1. First, brush the slow cooker bottom with olive oil.
2. Then roll up the dough and place it in the slow cooker.
3. Now flatten it in the shape of the pie crust.

5. Put the fish mixture over the pie crust and cover with foil.
6. Close the lid and cook the pie on Low for 7 hours.

Servings: 8

Preparation Time: 2 hours 40 minutes

Per Serving: 226 calories, 30.3g protein, 0.4g carbohydrates, 10.6g fat, 0.2g fiber, 86mg cholesterol, 782mg sodium, 536mg potassium.

Ingredients:

- 2 tablespoons lemon juice
- 1/2 cup of water
- 2 teaspoon salt
- 2 teaspoons ground cardamom
- 2-pounds trout fillet

Procedure:

1. In the shallow bowl mix butter, lemon juice, and salt.
2. Then sprinkle the trout fillet with ground cardamom and butter mixture.
3. Place the fish in the slow cooker and add water.
4. Cook the meal on High for 2.5 hours.

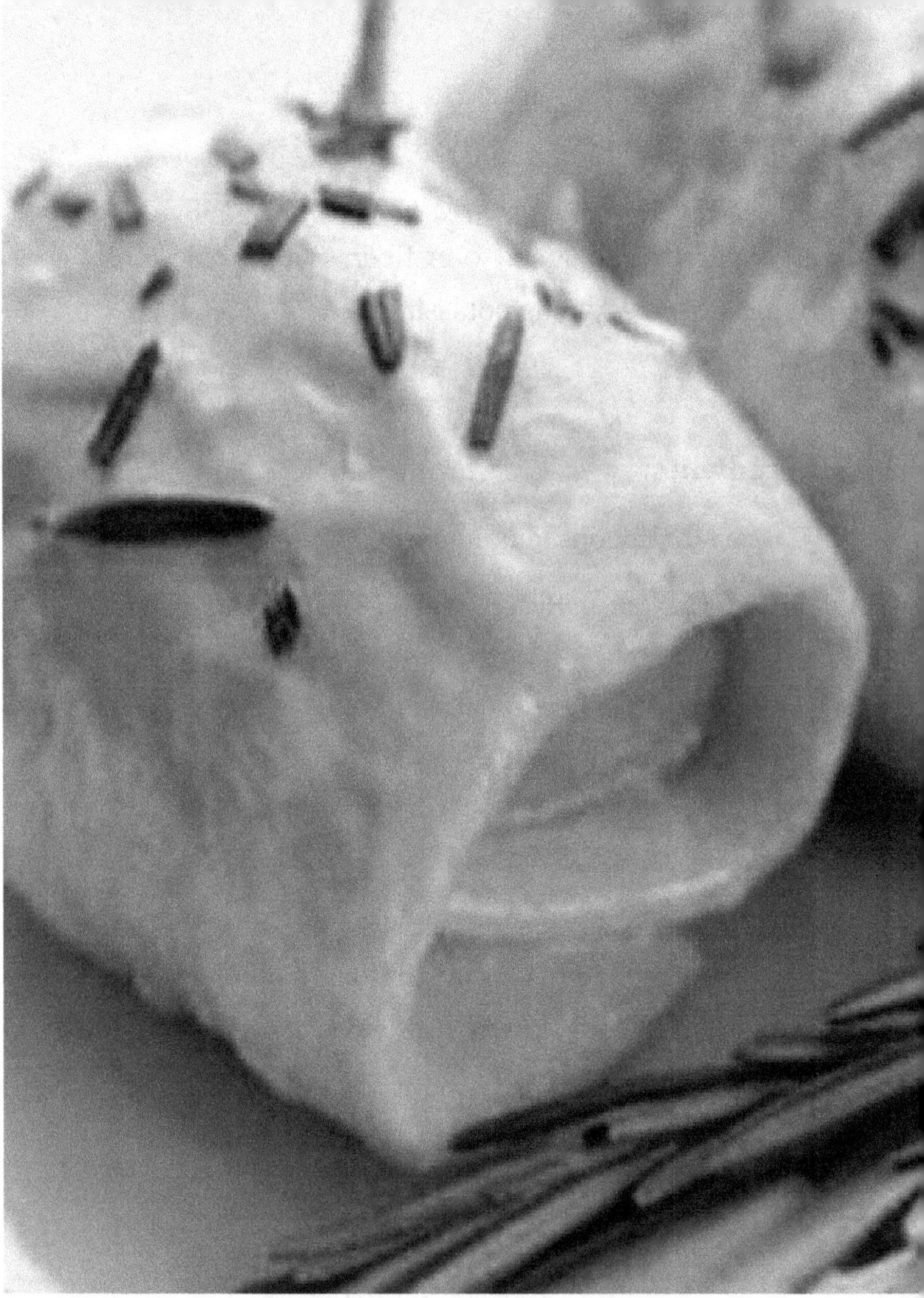

Servings: 4

Preparation Time: 2 hours 10 minutes

Per Serving: 149 calories, 27.6g protein, 1.5g carbohydrates, 2.9g fat, 1g fiber, 77mg cholesterol, 122mg sodium, 434mg potassium.

Ingredients:

- 2 tablespoons apple cider vinegar
- 10 tablespoons water
- 16 oz. sole fillet
- 2 tablespoons dried rosemary
- 2 tablespoons avocado oil

Procedure:

1. First, pour water in the slow cooker.
2. Then rub the sole fillet with dried rosemary and sprinkle with avocado oil and apple cider vinegar.
3. Now put the fish fillet in the slow cooker and cook it on High for 2 hours.

Servings: 4

Preparation Time: 1 hour 40 minutes

Per Serving: 121 calories, 21.3g protein, 0.1g carbohydrates, 3.4g fat, 0g fiber, 63mg cholesterol, 120mg sodium, 385mg potassium

Ingredients:

- 2 teaspoons olive oil
- 2 teaspoons lemon juice
- 12 oz haddock fillet
- 2 teaspoons dried cilantro
- 1/2 cup fish stock

Procedure:

1. First, heat the olive oil in the skillet well.
2. Then put the haddock fillet and roast it for 1 minute per side.
3. Now transfer the fillets in the slow cooker.
4. Add fish stock, cilantro, and lemon juice.
5. Cook the fish on high for 1.5 hours.

Servings: 8

Preparation Time: 3 hours 15 minutes

Per Serving: 166 calories, 20.8g protein, 1.2g carbohydrates, 8.8g fat, 0.5g fiber, 55mg cholesterol, 71mg sodium, 23mg potassium

Ingredients:

- 4 tablespoons sesame oil
- 1/2 cup of water
- 8 cod fillets
- 8 teaspoons mustard

Procedure:

1. First, mix mustard with sesame oil.
2. Then brush the cod fillets with mustard mixture and transfer in the slow cooker.
3. Now add water and cook the fish on low for 3 hours.

Servings: 4

Preparation Time: 2 hours 10 minutes

Per Serving: 444 calories, 23.9g protein, 0.5g carbohydrate: 38.7g fat, 0.1g fiber, 0mg cholesterol, 1mg sodium, 8mg potassium

Ingredients:

- 2 tablespoons olive oil
- 1 cup of water
- 2-pounds tuna fillet
- 2 teaspoons garlic powder

Procedure:

1. Sprinkle the tuna fillet with garlic powder.
2. Then pour olive oil in the skillet and heat it well.
3. Add the tuna and roast it for 1 minute per side.
4. Transfer the tuna in the slow cooker.
5. Add water and cook it on High for 2 hours.

Snacks

Servings: 12

Preparation Time: 6 hours

Per Serving: Calories 230 Fat 14.8 g Carbohydrates 8.9 g Sugar 1.1 g Protein 15.7 g Cholesterol 48 mg

Ingredients:

- 16 Oz cream cheese, softened
- 28 Oz can artichoke hearts, drained and chopped
- 20 Oz frozen spinach, thawed and drained
- 1/8 Tsp garlic powder
- 4 Tbsp water
- 4 Cups cottage cheese
- 2 Tsp salt

Procedure:

1. Firstly, add spinach, cream cheese, cottage cheese, water, and artichoke hearts to a crock pot and stir well
2. Then, season with garlic powder and salt.
3. Finally, cover and cook on low for 6 hours.
4. Now, stir well and serve.

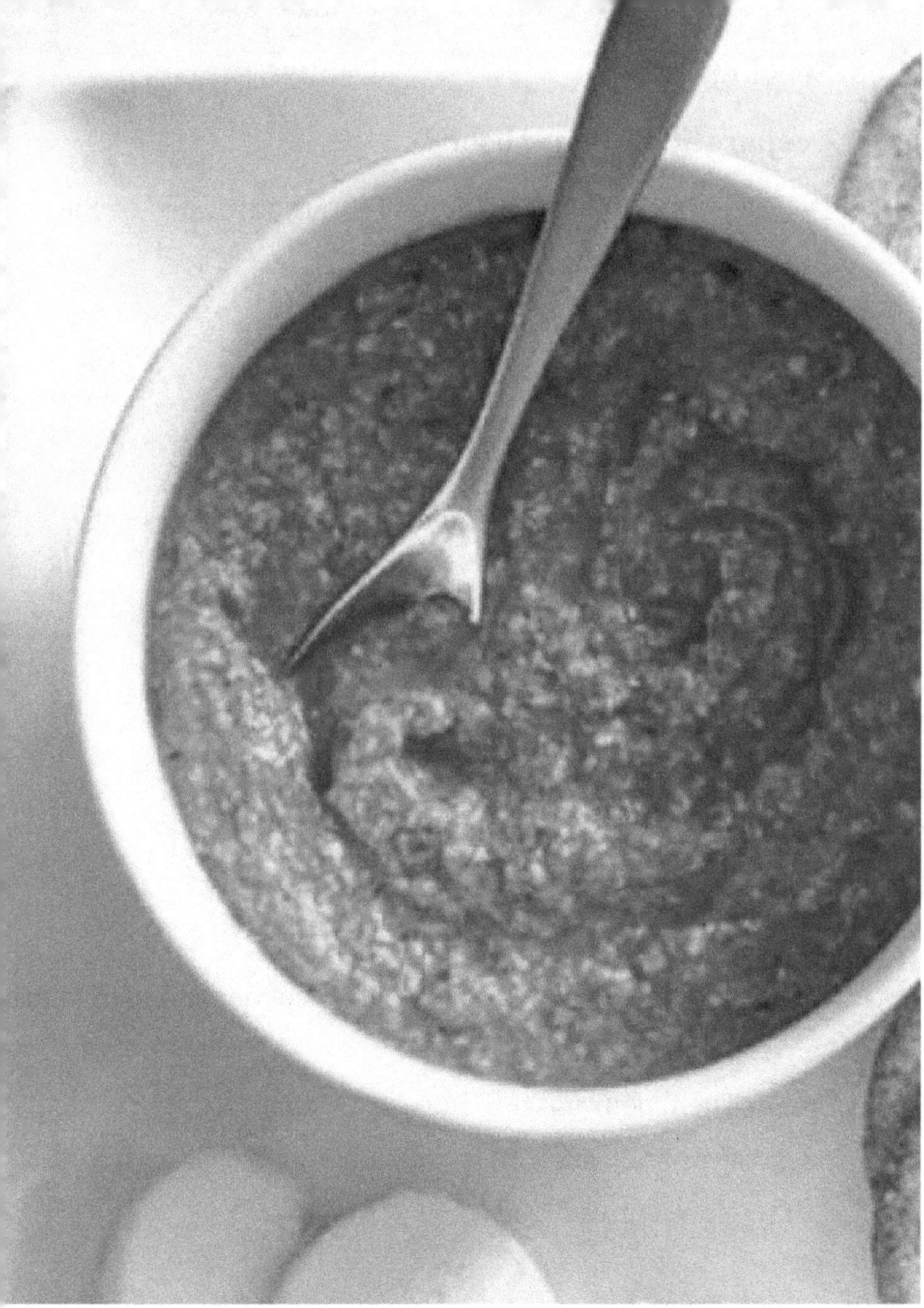

Servings: 10

Preparation Time: 1 hour

Per Serving: Calories 47 Fat 4.5 g Carbohydrates 1 g Sugar 0.1 g Protein 1 g Cholesterol 13 mg

Ingredients:

- 16 Oz cream cheese
- 1/8 Cup sun-dried tomatoes
- 2 Tbsp mayonnaise
- 6 Garlic cloves
- 1/8 Tsp white pepper
- 2 Tsp pine nuts, toasted
- 3/4 Oz fresh basil

Procedure:

1. Firstly, add all ingredients to a blender and blend until smooth.
2. Then, pour mixture into a crock pot.
3. Cover and cook on low for 1 hour.
4. Now, stir well and serve.

Servings: 6

Preparation Time: 4 hours

Per Serving: Calories 95 Fat 8.5 g Carbohydrates 4.3 g Sugar 1.6 g Protein 1.4 g Cholesterol 14 mg

Ingredients:

- 8 Onions, sliced
- 4 Tbsp olive oil
- 4 Tbsp butter
- 1 Cup mozzarella cheese
- 16 Oz sour cream
- Pepper
- Salt

Procedure:

1. Firstly, add oil, butter, and onions to a crock pot.
2. Then, cover and cook on high for 4 hours.
3. Transfer onion mixture to a blender with the sour cream, pepper, and salt and blend until creamy.

4. Return onion dip to the crock pot.
5. Finally, add mozzarella cheese and stir well. Cook on low for 30 minutes longer.
6. Stir well and serve.

Servings: 8

Preparation Time: 3 hours

Per Serving: Calories 253 Fat 21.6 g Carbohydrates 14.5 g Sugar 4.1 g Protein 5.1 g Cholesterol 31 mg

Ingredients:

- 2 lb green beans, rinsed and trimmed
- 1 Cup almonds, sliced and toasted
- 1 Cup vegetable stock
- 1/8 Cup butter, melted
- 12 Oz onion, sliced
- 2 Tbsp olive oil
- 1/2 Tsp pepper
- 1 Tsp salt

Procedure:

1. Firstly, heat the olive oil in a pan over medium heat.
2. Add onion to the pan and sauté until softened.
3. Then, transfer sautéed onion to a crock pot.

5. Finally, cover and cook on low for 3 hours.
6. Now, top with toasted almonds and serve.

Servings: 8

Preparation Time: 3 hours

Per Serving: Calories 79 Fat 3.9 g Carbohydrates 11.4 g Sugar 6.9 g Protein 1.7 g Cholesterol 0 mg

Ingredients:

- 2 Cup cherry tomatoes, halved
- 6 Bell peppers, cut into strips
- 2 Onions, sliced
- 2 Tsp paprika
- 2 Tbsp olive oil
- Pepper and salt

Procedure:

1. Firstly, add onion, bell peppers, oil, smoked paprika, pepper, and salt to a crock pot and stir well.
2. Then, cover and cook on high for 1 1/2 hours.
3. Add cherry tomatoes and cook for 2 hours longer.
4. Now, stir well and serve.

Servings: 4

Preparation Time: 5 hours

Per Serving: calories 158, fat 13.3, fiber 3.9, carbs 8.9, protein 3.3

Ingredients:

- 20 Oz cauliflower
- 2 Teaspoons curry paste
- 2 Teaspoons curry powder
- 1 Teaspoon dried cilantro
- 2 Oz butter
- ¾ Cup water
- 1/2 Cup chicken stock

Procedure:

1. Firstly, chop the cauliflower roughly and sprinkle it with the curry powder and dried cilantro.
2. Then, place the chopped cauliflower in the slow cooker
3. Mix the curry paste with the water.

5. Add butter and close the lid.
6. Cook the cauliflower for 5 hours on Low.
7. Finally, strain ½ of the liquid off and discard. Transfer the cauliflower to serving bowls.
8. Now, serve it!

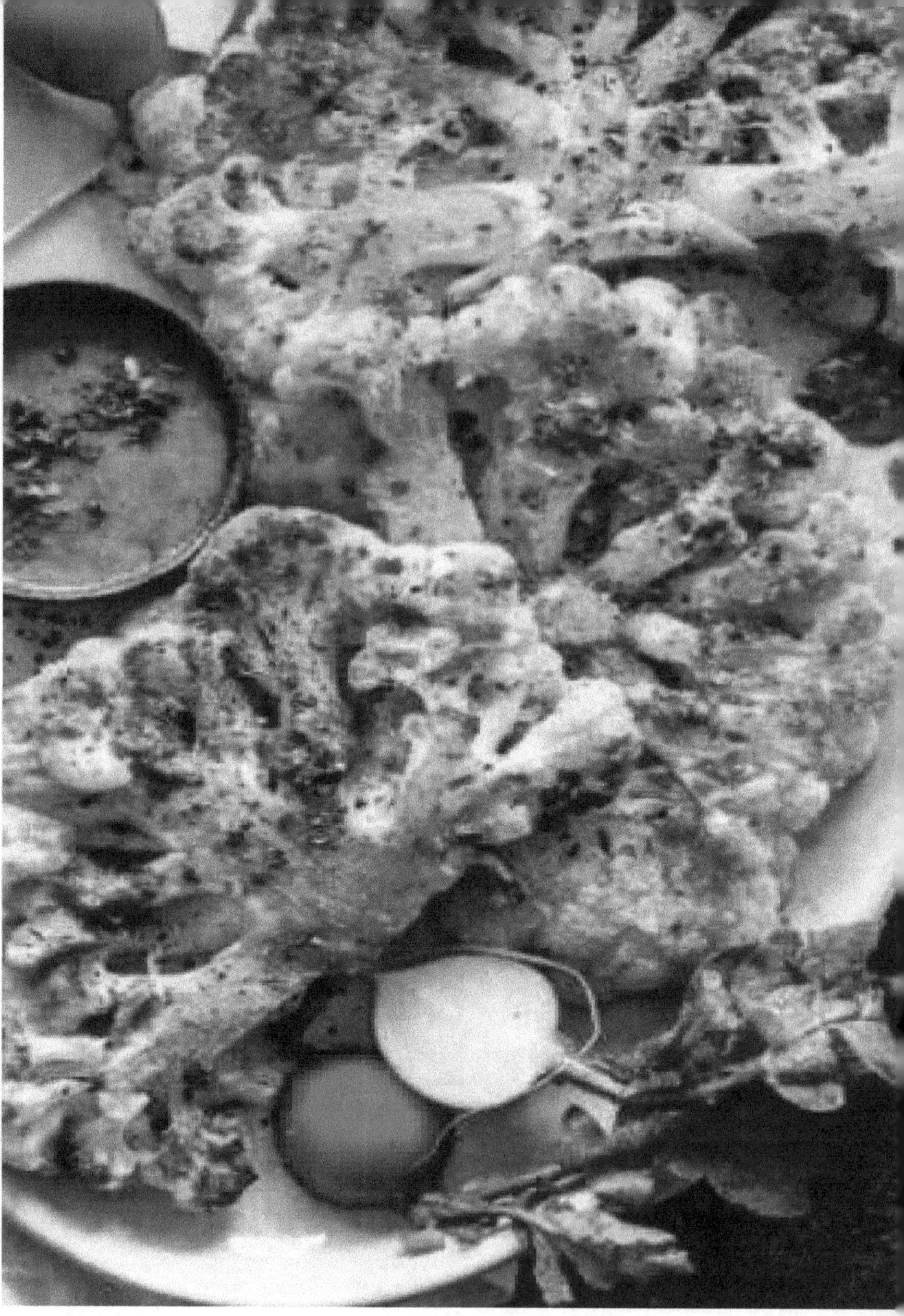

Servings: 8

Preparation Time: 3 hours

Per Serving: calories 129, fat 11.7, fiber 2.7, carbs 5.8, protein 2.2

Ingredients:

- 28 Oz cauliflower head
- 2 Teaspoons minced garlic
- 8 Tablespoons butter
- 8 Tablespoons water 1 teaspoon paprika

Procedure:

1. Firstly, wash the cauliflower head carefully and slice it into the medium steaks.
2. Mix up together the butter, minced garlic, and paprika.
3. Then, rub the cauliflower steaks with the butter mixture.
4. Pour the water in the slow cooker.

7. Now, transfer the cooked cauliflower steaks to a platter and serve them immediately!

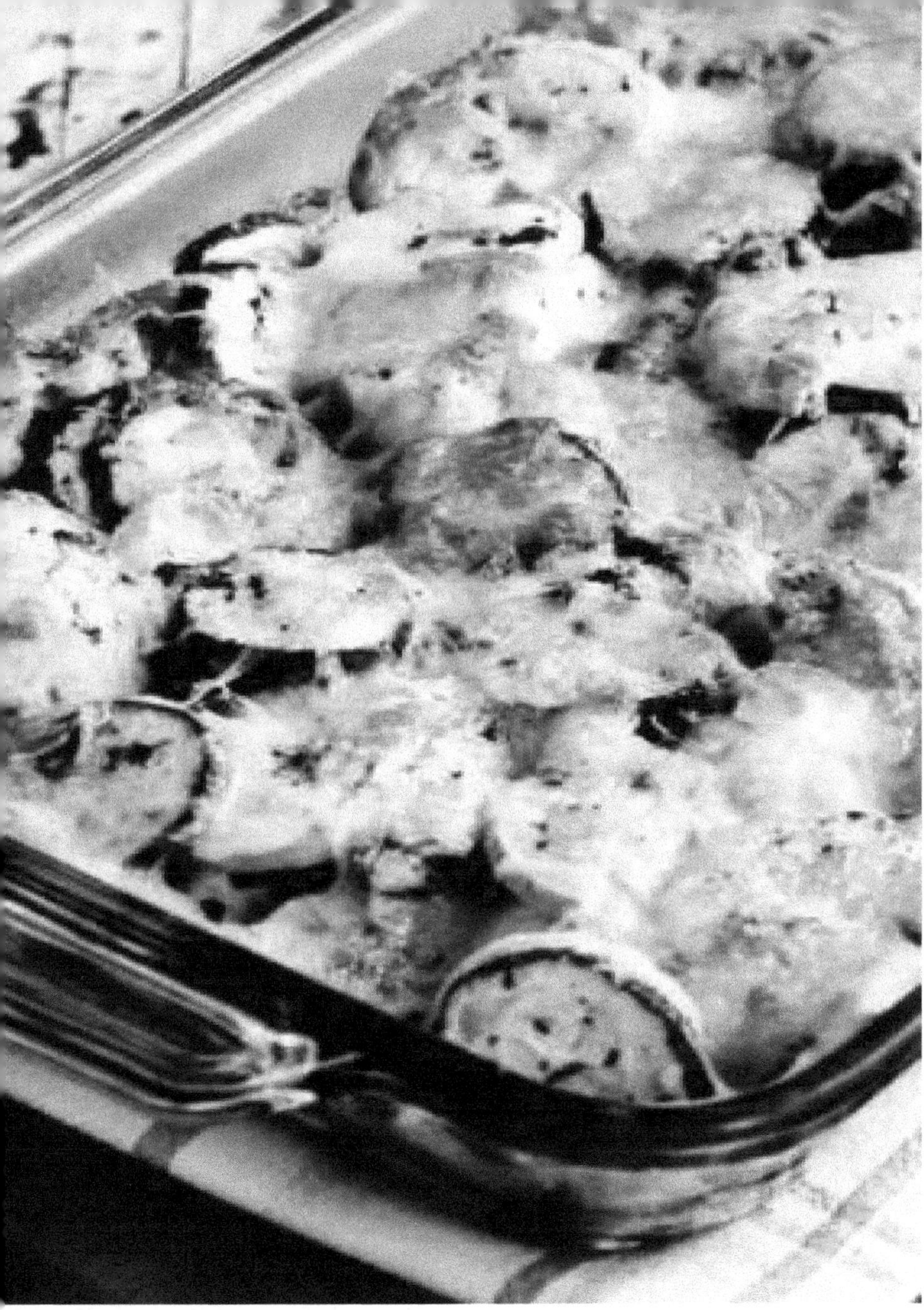

Servings: 6

Preparation Time: 5 hours

Per Serving: calories 229, fat 19.6, fiber 1.8, carbs 5.9, protein 10.9

Ingredients:

- 2 Zucchini, sliced
- 6 Oz Parmesan, grated
- 2 Teaspoons ground black pepper
- 2 Tablespoons butter
- 1 Cup almond milk

Procedure:

1. Firstly, sprinkle the sliced zucchini with the ground black pepper.
2. Then, chop the butter and place it in the slow cooker.
3. Transfer the sliced zucchini to the slow cooker to make the bottom layer.

5. Sprinkle the zucchini with the grated cheese and close the lid.

6. Cook the gratin for 5 hours on Low.

7. Finally, let the gratin cool until room temperature.

8. Now, serve it!

Servings: 4

Preparation Time: 5 hours

Per Serving: calories 107, fat 5.4, fiber 5.6, carbs 10, protein 6.8

Ingredients:

- 1/2 Tablespoon butter
- 1/2 Teaspoon minced garlic
- 1 Eggplants, chopped
- 1/2 Teaspoon salt
- 1/2 Tablespoon dried parsley
- 2 Oz Parmesan, grated
- 2 Tablespoons water
- 2 Teaspoon chili flakes

Procedure:

1. Firstly, mix the dried parsley, chili flakes, and salt together.
2. Then, sprinkle the chopped eggplants with the spice mixture and stir well.

4. Add the water and minced garlic.

5. Add the butter and sprinkle with the grated Parmesan.

6. Finally, close the lid and cook the gratin for 5 hours on Low.

7. Open the lid and cool the gratin for 10 minutes.

8. Now, serve it.

Servings: 8

Preparation Time: 7 hour

Per Serving: calories 190, fat 17, fiber 5.6, carbs 10, protein 2.5

Ingredients:

- 2 Eggplant, peeled
- 2 Jalapeno pepper
- 2 Teaspoon curry powder
- 1 Teaspoon salt
- 2 Teaspoons paprika
- ¾ Teaspoon ground nutmeg
- 4 Tablespoons butter
- ¾ Cup almond milk
- 1 Teaspoon dried dill

Procedure:

1. Firstly, chop the eggplant into small pieces.
2. Place the eggplant in the slow cooker.

4. Finally, sprinkle the vegetables with the curry powder, salt, paprika, ground nutmeg, and dried dill.

5. Add almond milk and butter.

6. Close the lid and cook the vegetables for 7 hours on Low.

7. Cool the vegetables and then blend them until smooth with a hand blender.

8. Now, transfer the cooked eggplant mash into the bowls and serve!

Servings: 12

Preparation Time: 7 hours

Per Serving: 235 calories, 10.9g protein, 45.9g carbohydrates, 0.7g fat, 10.8g fiber, 0mg cholesterol, 12mg sodium, 432mg potassium.

Ingredients:

- 2 Teaspoon cumin seeds
- 2 Cup red lentils
- 1 Teaspoon fennel seeds
- 10 Cups of water
- 1 Cup tomatoes, chopped
- 1/2 Cup onion, diced
- 1 Teaspoon ground ginger
- 2 Cups of rice

Procedure:

1. Firstly, put ingredients from the list above in the slow cooker.
2. Then, carefully stir the mixture and close the lid.
3. Now, cook the tomato dal on low for 7 hours.

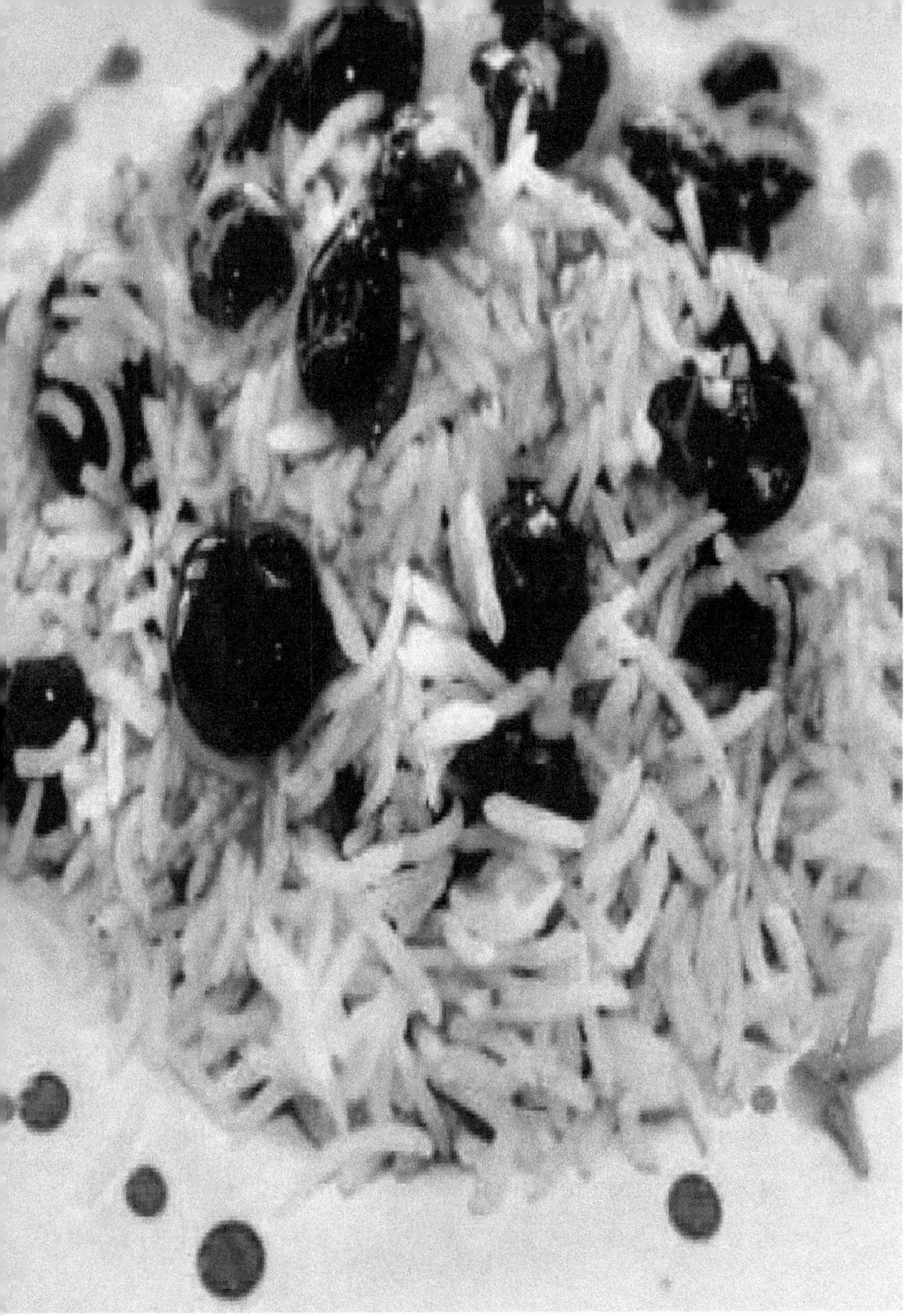

Servings: 8

Preparation Time: 6 hours

Per Serving: 324 calories, 20.9g protein, 57.4g carbohydrates, 2.2g fat, 14.2g fiber, 0mg cholesterol, 26mg sodium, 1274mg potassium

Ingredients:

- 4 Cups red kidney beans, soaked
- 2 Cayenne pepper, chopped
- 1 Teaspoon garlic powder
- 2 Teaspoon onion powder
- 16 Cups of water
- 2 Teaspoon coconut oil

Procedure:

1. Firstly, put all ingredients in the slow cooker.
2. Cook the mixture for 6 hours on high.
3. Then, transfer the cooked bean mixture in the blender and pulse for 15 seconds.
4. Now, transfer the meal in the bowls

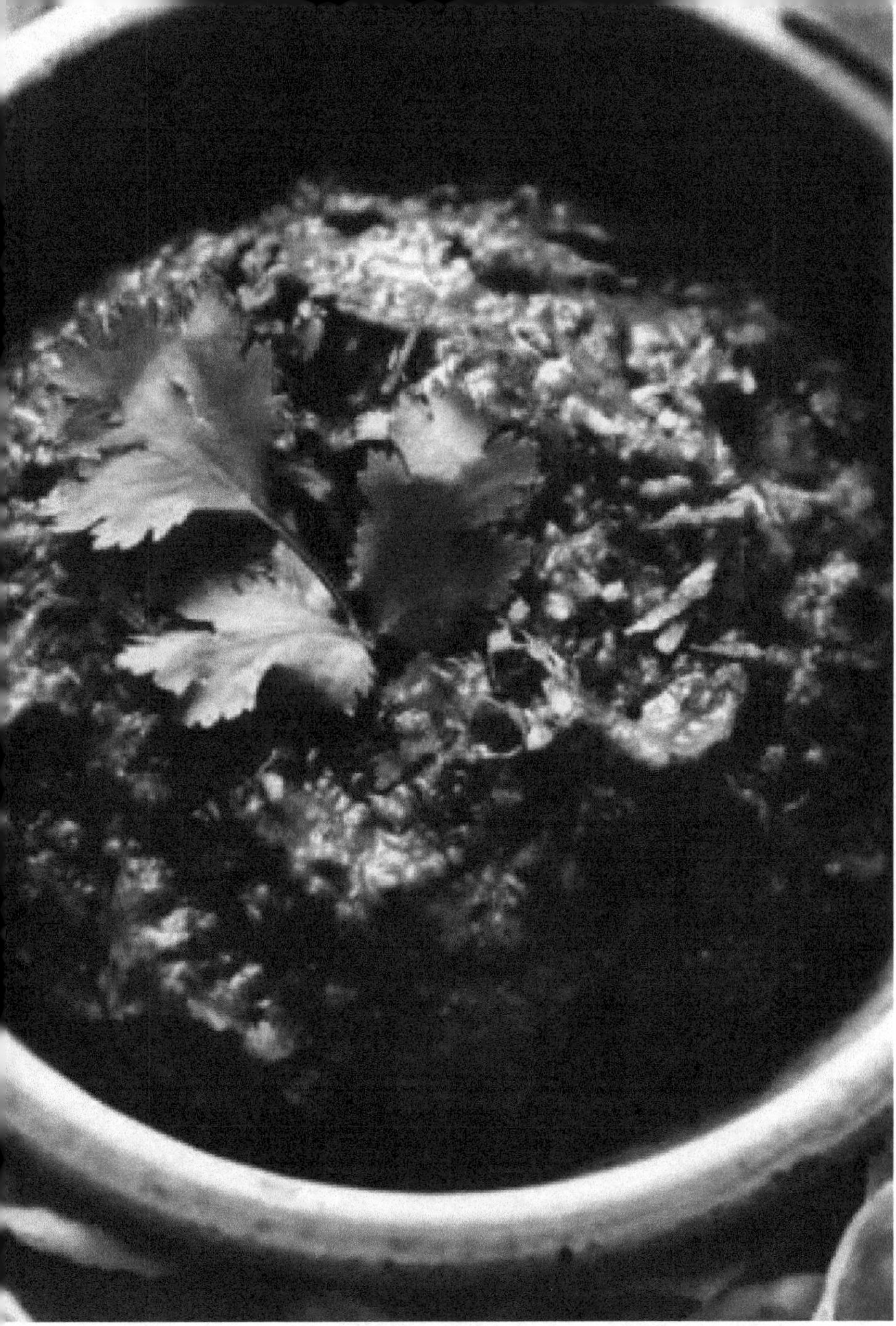

Servings: 12

Preparation Time: 20 minutes

Per Serving: 134 calories, 7.2g protein, 10.8g carbohydrates 7.8g fat, 3.7g fiber, 169mg cholesterol, 87mg sodium, 361mg potassium.

Ingredients:

- 12 Eggs
- 4 Oz chilies, canned, chopped
- 2 Cup tomatoes, canned
- 2 Onions, diced
- 2 Tablespoon butter
- 2 Teaspoon olive oil
- 1 Cup bell pepper, chopped
- 1 Cup of water
- 2 Teaspoon smoked paprika

1. Firstly, mix chilies, tomatoes, onion, olive oil, bell pepper, water, and smoked paprika in the slow cooker.
2. Then, close the lid and cook the mixture on high for 2 hours.
3. Meanwhile, melt the butter in the skillet.
4. Crack the eggs in the hot oil and roast them for 4 minutes or until the eggs are solid.
5. Finally, transfer the eggs in the plates.
6. Now, top them with cooked tomato mixture from the slow cooker.

Dessert

Servings: 12

Preparation Time: 2 hours

Per Serving: Calories 59 Fat 0.2 g Carbohydrates 15 g Sugar 11.7 g Protein 0.3 g Cholesterol 0 mg

Ingredients:

- 6 lb apples, peeled, cored, and sliced
- 4 Cinnamon sticks
- 2 Tbsp fresh lemon juice
- 1/2 Cup water

Procedure:

1. Firstly, add all ingredients to a crock pot and stir well.
2. Cover and cook on high for 2 hours.
3. Then, discard cinnamon sticks and mash the apples with a potato masher until you have the desired consistency.

Servings: 12

Preparation Time: 8 hours

Per Serving: Calories 41 Fat 0.3 g Carbohydrates 9.7 g Suga
9.4 g Protein 1 g Cholesterol 0 mg

Ingredients:

- 8 lb frozen peaches, thawed
- 1/2 Tsp ground cloves
- 1 Tsp ground ginger
- 2 tsp fresh lemon juice
- 1 Cup Swerve

Procedure:

1. Firstly, add peaches to a blender and blend until smooth and creamy.
2. Transfer blended peaches to a crock pot along with Swerve and stir well.

5. Now, allow to cool completely and store in a container in the refrigerator.

Servings: 7

Preparation Time: 24 hours

Per Serving: Calories 10 Fat 0 g Carbohydrates 2 g Sugar 1 Protein 0 g Cholesterol 0 mg

Ingredients:

- 2 Large ham bone
- 2 Tsp black peppercorns
- 2 Bay leaf
- 2 Thyme sprig
- 2 Garlic clove, peeled
- 4 Carrots, cut in half
- 2 Celery stalk, cut in half
- 2 Onions, peeled and quartered

1. First, add all ingredients to a crock pot.
2. Fill crock pot with cold water.
3. Then, cover and cook on low for 24 hours.
4. Now, strain the stock into a container and store in the refrigerator.

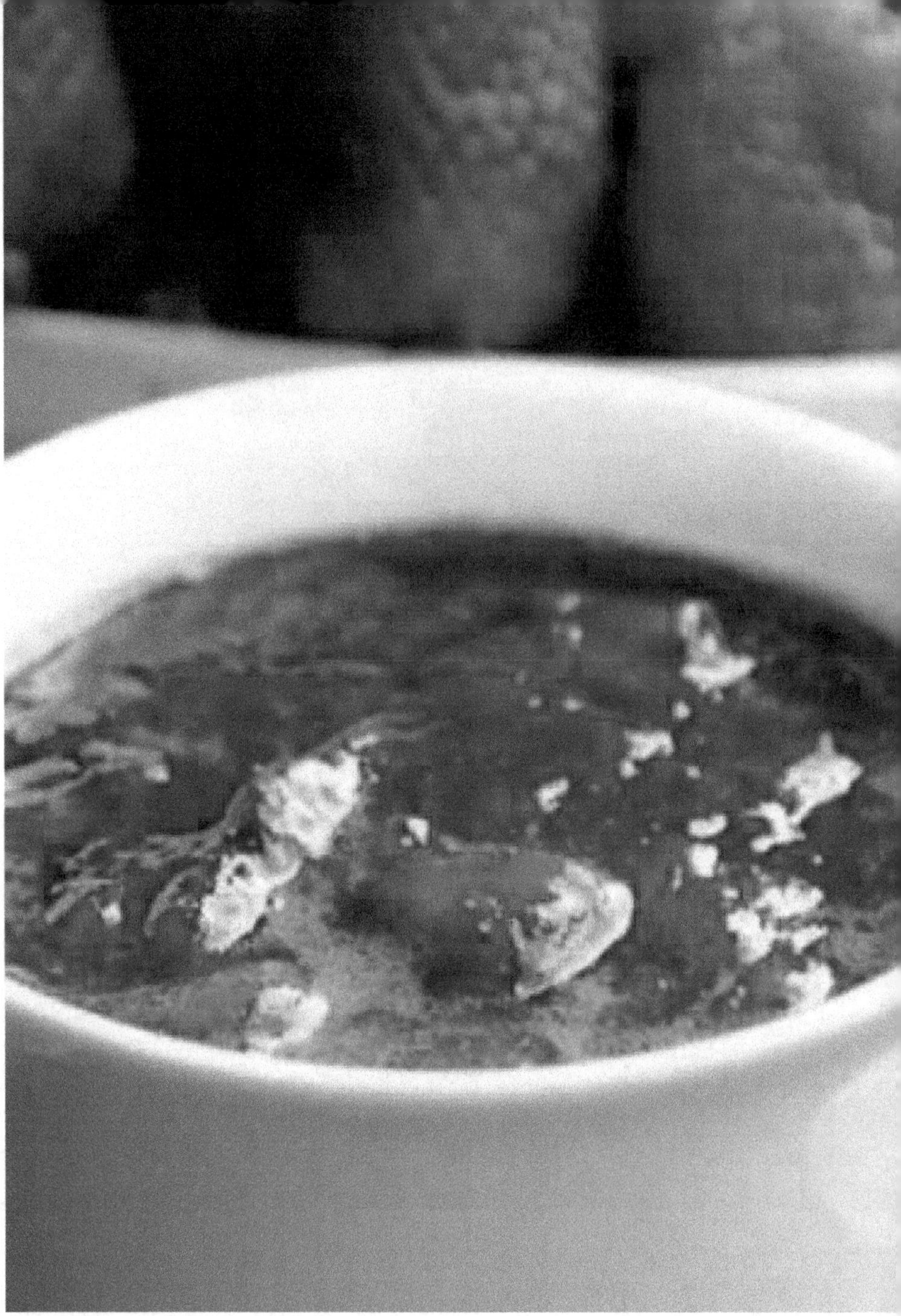

Servings: 8

Preparation Time: 2 hours

Per Serving: Calories 38 Fat 0.4 g Carbohydrates 8.9 g Sugar 5.6 g Protein 0.8 g Cholesterol 0 mg

Ingredients:

- 2 lb strawberries, hulled and chopped
- 2 Tbsp fresh lemon juice
- 1/2 Cup Swerve
- Pinch of salt

Procedure:

1. Firstly, add strawberries, Swerve, and salt to a crock pot.
2. Cover and cook on low for 2 hours.
3. Then, add lemon juice and stir well.
4. Now, once sauce has cooled completely, pour it into a container and store in the refrigerator.

Servings: 8

Preparation Time: 4 hours

Per Serving: Calories 61 Fat 0.3 g Carbohydrates 16.1 g Sugar 11.5 g Protein 0.5 g Cholesterol 0 mg

Ingredients:

- 3 lb apples
- 2 Tsp cinnamon
- 4 Tbsp water
- 8 Oz blueberries

Procedure:

1. Firstly, add all ingredients to a crock pot and stir to mix.
2. Cover and cook on low for 4 hours.
3. Then, blend the sauce using an immersion blender unt the desired consistency.
4. Now, once sauce has cooled completely, store in a container in the refrigerator.

Servings: 4

Preparation Time: 2 hours

Per Serving: Calories 162, Fat 2, Fiber 2, Carbs 4, Protein 5

Ingredients:

- 2 Cups plums, pitted and halved
- 2 Cups rhubarb, sliced
- 2 Cups coconut cream
- 1 Teaspoon vanilla extract
- 1 Cup sugar
- 1 Tablespoon lemon juice 1 teaspoon almond extract

Procedure:

1. Firstly, in your slow cooker, mix the plums with the rhubarb, cream and the other ingredients, toss, put the lid on and cook on High for 2 hours.
2. Then, divide the mix into bowls and serve.

Servings: 8

Preparation Time: 1 hour

Per Serving: Calories 152, f At 3, Fiber 5, Carbs 12, Protein

Ingredients:

- 8 Pears
- Juice and Zest of 1 lemon
- 52 Ounces grape juice
- 22 Ounces currant jelly
- 8 Garlic cloves ½ vanilla bean
- 8 Peppercorns 2 rosemary springs

Procedure:

1. First, put the jelly, grape juice, lemon zest, lemon juice vanilla, peppercorns, rosemary and pears in your slow cooker, cover and cook on High for 1 hour and 30 minutes.
2. Then, divide everything between plates and serve.

Servings: 4

Preparation Time: 2 hours

Per Serving: Calories 172, Fat 2, Fiber 3, Carbs 4, Protein 5

Ingredients:

- 2 Cup cream cheese, soft
- 1 Cup Greek yogurt
- 4 Eggs, whisked
- 1 Teaspoon baking soda
- 2 Cup almonds, chopped
- 1 Tablespoon sugar
- 1 Teaspoon almond extract ½ teaspoon cinnamon powder

Procedure:

1. Firstly, in your slow cooker, mix the cream cheese with the yogurt, eggs and the other ingredients, whisk, put the lid on and cook on Low for 2 hours.
2. Now, divide the pudding into bowls and serve.

Servings: 12

Preparation Time: 2 hours

Per Serving: Calories 152, Fat 4, Fiber 4 , Carbs 6, Protein 4

Ingredients:

- 2 Tablespoon butter
- 14 Ounces long grain rice
- 8 Ounces water
- 32 ounces milk
- 6 Ounces sugar
- 2 Eggs
- 1 Tablespoon cream 1 teaspoon vanilla extract

Procedure:

1. First, in your slow cooker, mix butter with rice, water, milk, sugar, egg, cream and vanilla, stir, cover and cook on High for 2 hours.
2. Now, stir pudding one more time, divide into bowls and serve.

95

Tasty Cinnamon Plum Jam

Servings: 12

Preparation Time: 6 hours

Per Serving: 71 calories, 0.4g protein, 18.2g carbohydrates, 0.1g fat, 1.2g fiber, 0mg cholesterol, 4mg sodium, 91mg potassium.

Ingredients:

- 8 Cups plums, pitted, halved
- 2 Tablespoons ground cinnamon
- 1 Cup brown sugar
- 1 Teaspoon vanilla extract

Procedure:

1. First, put all ingredients in the slow cooker and gently mix.
2. Then, close the lid and cook it on Low for 6 hours.

Tempting Tarragon Peach Confiture

Servings: 12

Preparation Time: 2.5 hours

Per Serving: 73 calories, 0.3g protein, 19.1g carbohydrates, 0.1g fat, 0.4g fiber, 0mg cholesterol, 0mg sodium, 52mg potassium.

Ingredients:

- 2-Pound peaches, pitted, halved
- 1 Cup of sugar
- 2 Teaspoons lemon zest, grated
- 2 Teaspoons dried tarragon
- 1/3 Cup water

1. Firstly, put all ingredients in the slow cooker and close the lid.
2. Then, cook the dessert on high for 2.5 hours.
3. Now, cool the cooked confiture well.

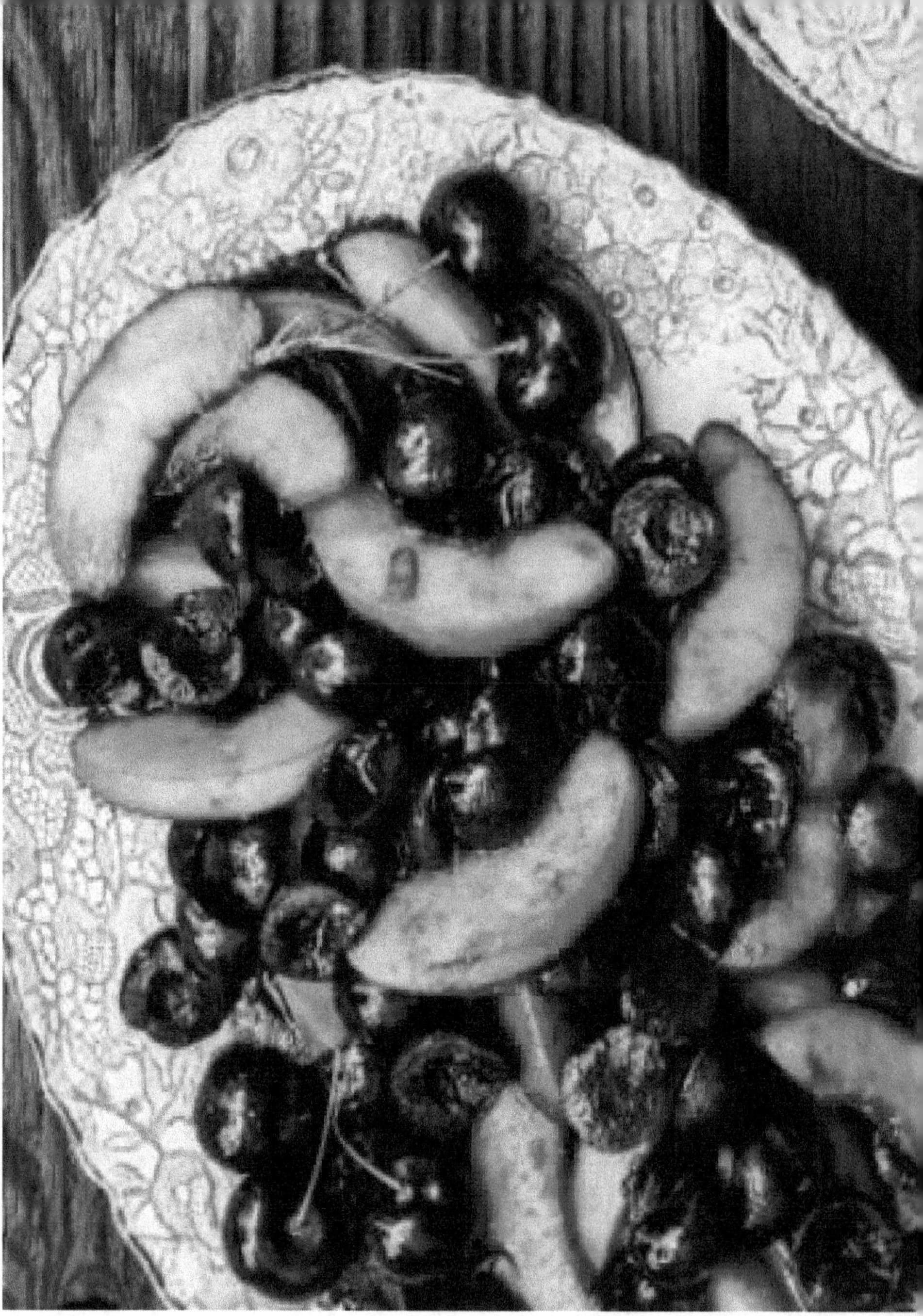

Servings: 12

Preparation Time: 3 hours

Per Serving: : 93 calories, 0.7g protein, 23.9g carbohydrates, 0.3g fat, 1.4g fiber, 0mg cholesterol, 11mg sodium, 117mg potassium.

Ingredients:

- 2 Cup apricots, pitted, chopped
- 1 Cup cherries, pitted
- 2 Cups strawberries
- 1/2 Cup blackberries
- 1 Cup of sugar
- 16 Cups of water

Procedure:

1. Firstly, put all ingredients in the slow cooker.
2. Then, cook compote on High for 3 hours.
3. Now, cool it and serve with ice cubes.

Servings: 12

Preparation Time: 8 hours

Per Serving: 157 calories, 1.4g protein, 40.2g carbohydrates 0.3g fat, 2.8g fiber, 0mg cholesterol, 6mg sodium, 436mg potassium.

Ingredients:

- 4-Pounds rhubarb, chopped
- 2 Cups of sugar
- 2 Teaspoons lime zest, grated
- 1/2 Cup of water

Procedure:

1. Firstly, put all ingredients in the slow cooker.
2. Cook the jam on Low for 8 hours.
3. Then, transfer it in the glass jars and cool well.

CPSIA information can be obtained
at www.ICGtesting.com
Printed in the USA
BVHW091113170521
607543BV00006B/796

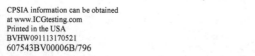

9 781802 947670